Herbs for Women's Health
By: Alize Priest

Copyright © 2023 by: Alize Priest
Publisher: Poitier Wordsmith Academy…
Poitier Publishing Company
All rights reserved. No part of this book may be reproduced or transmitted in any form or by any means, electronic or mechanical, including photocopying, recording, or by any information storage and retrieval system, without permission in writing from the author or publisher.

ISBN: 9798398647686
Printed in the United States of America.

Caution...

This book was written by an 18-year-old who has experienced a number of conditions and has found natural herbs that can address these common issues, again naturally.

I am not a doctor, yet so... please do not use these herbs as substitution for any prescribed medication.

Any treatment should be discussed with a medical professional. It is just my desire to give women affordable and healthy suggestions for improving their health state as women. Each herb can be researched online and there are a number of You-Tube informational videos about each of them. Thank you for finding interest in my work and in your own health journey...

Dedication…

I dedicate this book to women who suffer with difficulty having babies, suffer from difficulty carrying a baby to full term, or suffer with types of infertility and health issues like endometriosis, hormone imbalance, PCOS (Polycystic Ovary Syndrome), failure to ovulate, or problems with periods.

I wanted to make this book for women who suffer with infertility because I noticed nowadays there are more and more women saying that they have trouble getting pregnant or being able to carry a baby to full term and I also dedicate this book to women who have painful periods. At one time I used to also have very painful periods until I tried these herbs. My pain used to be so bad I was throwing up, shaking, had headaches, I was bloated, and more… so if you suffer from any of these symptoms or issues…

This book is dedicated you!

Table of Contents

Red Raspberry leaf 8-9

Maca root 10-11

Fenugreek 12-13

Ashwaganda 14-15

Sea buckthorn 16-17

Dong quai 18-19

Black cohosh 20-21

Dandelion 22

Slippery elm 23

Health Plan 24-25

I am Alize 27

Herb 1: Red Raspberry leaf

Red raspberry leaf is good for women and has been traditionally used to support the female reproductive system. This leaf could help reduce PMS, Pre-menstrual symptom(s) such as cramping and regulating periods for women who have irregular periods. These are the elements of the female reproductive system that it supports along with directions on how to use the leaf:

- Red raspberry strengthens your uterus if you drink it.
- To minimize period cramps drink it up to 3-4 days before your period.
- It also supports fertility for women who have problems with their fertility.
- It assists if you just want a "boost."
- Another common thing that women use Red raspberry leaf tea for is for labor when they are about to give birth because it decreases the time of labor.

Note: Though It strengthens your uterus for improving your labor experience, *pregnant ladies do not take it until it is time to push that baby out.* It is not good to take in early pregnancy because it could cause some problems.

I also recommend it for my older ladies… it helps with menopause, making that transition much easier.

If you are thinking about drinking this tea, drink it only 2 times a day one in the afternoon and one in the evening.

Red Raspberry Leaf

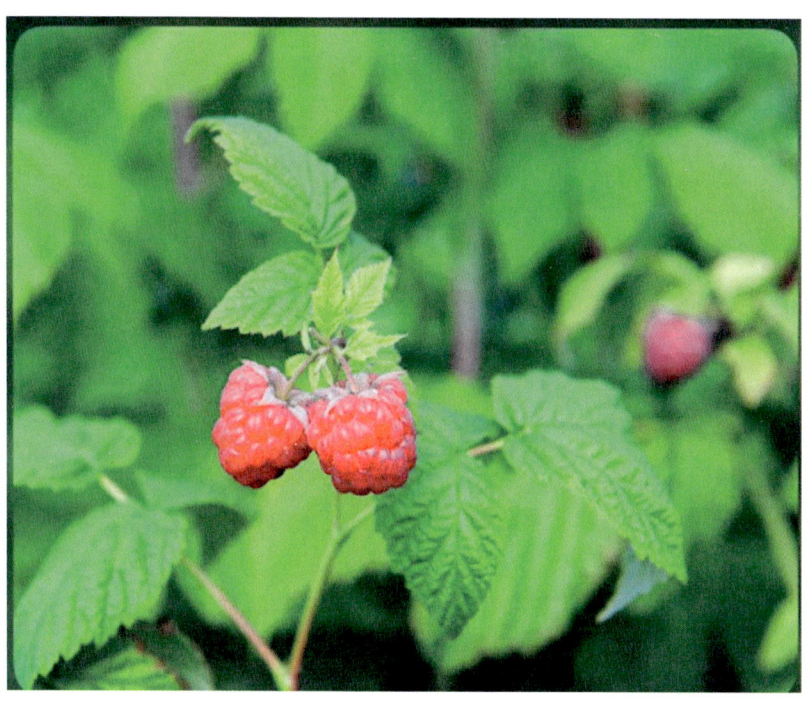

Maca Root

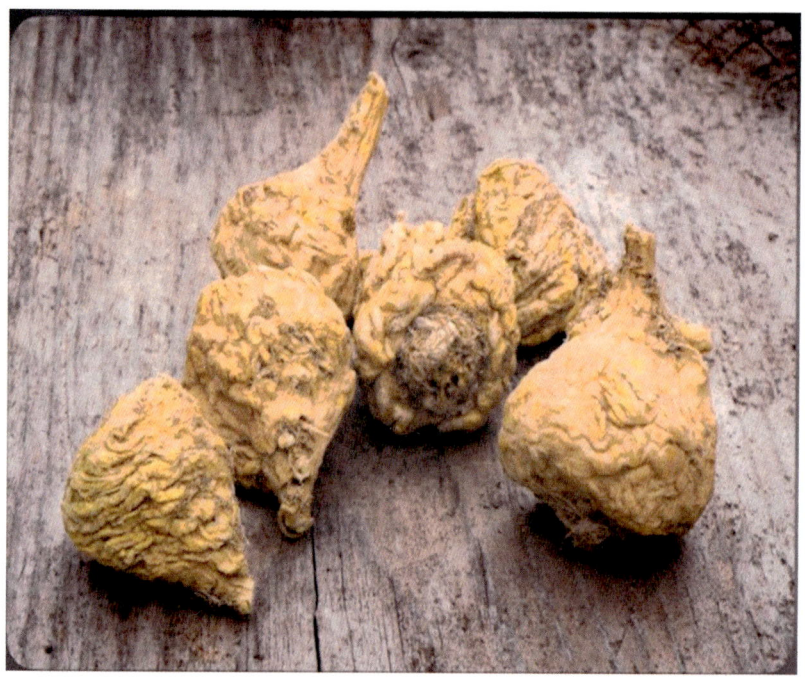

Herb 2: Maca Root

Maca root is a nutritionally dense superfood that has been used by women for numerous issues. Maca root can be helpful to women because it helps with increasing skin health, a much-needed boost in our present environmental state. You will age beautifully with the aid of the Maca root. Maca root has also been known for the following things with women:

Herb 2: Maca Root continued

- To boost your fertility naturally, so I would be careful taking this if you do not want to have multiple babies running around!
- Maca root gives you mental clarity so if you have trouble keeping things straight... try Maca root.
- It addresses some memory loss.
- If you have a tough time focusing on things, Maca root can be taken to assist with bringing focus back.
- Also, it has been associated with aiding women in keeping regular periods.
- If you have certain thyroid issues like myself, I struggle with hypothyroidism, it is helpful with those conditions.
- As we discussed fertility, it also will boost your libido those of you struggling with certain things in the bedroom.
- Maca root can be used to *grow your hair*.
- Maca root is good for those struggling with depression; it is great for reducing that and if you want to take Maca root for this symptom, I recommend taking it as a pill.

Herb 3: Fenugreek

Fenugreek does wonders for a woman's body. The main uses are:
- It is well known to help lower blood sugar in people with diabetes.
- It may also help regulate cholesterol.
- It may help you relieve menstrual cramps.
- Another reason a lot of people take this herb is because it helps you with *wetness down there* (moisture in the vaginal region).
- Ladies… it helps you *smell sweet*; even your sweat is going to *smell sweet*.
- It could increase the sex drive so be careful "girlies."

Note: Some of these herbs make you *act up*

For my mommies out there, this could help increase your milk flow as well, so I recommend taking this as a pill or in powered form.

Fenugreek

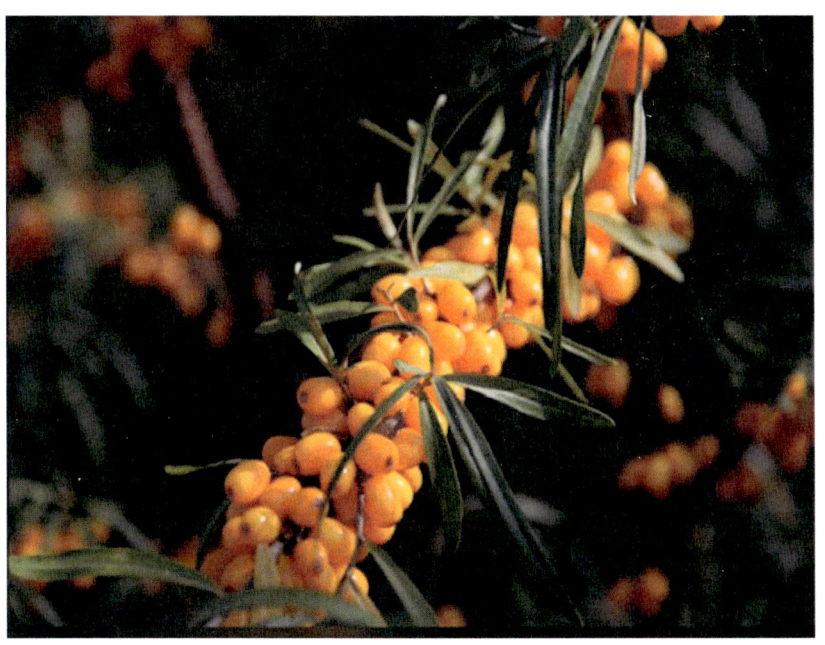

Ashwaganda

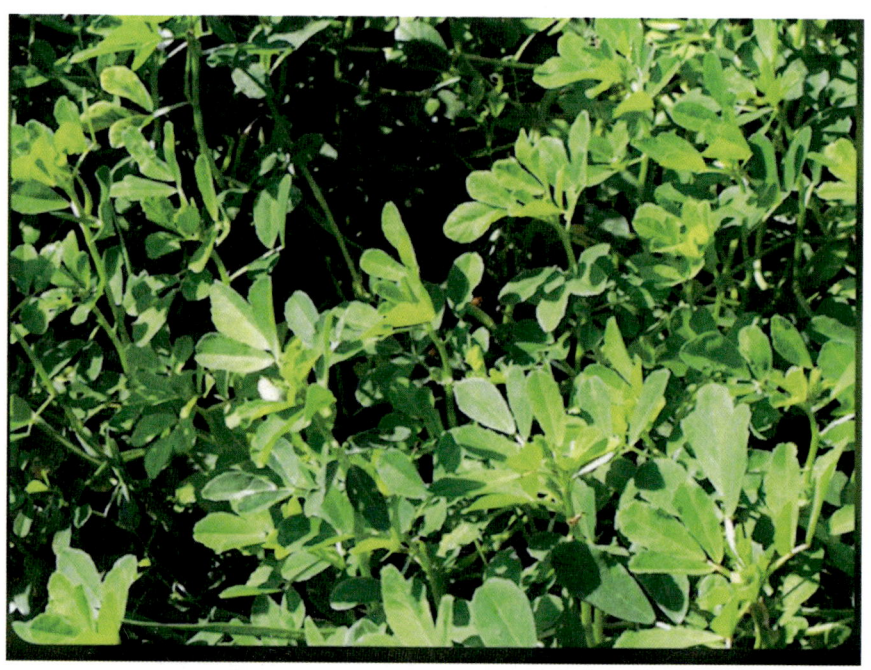

Herb 4: Ashwaganda

Ashwaganda is a great herb for women because it is a natural stress reliever, so it calms you down physically and mentally. Nothing is going to bother you so on those days where you are just not *feeling it* or you know it is going to be a stressful day, this is the herb to take. Here are the health aids this herb offers:

Herb 4: Ashwaganda continued

- This herb improves cognitive functions.
- It helps you focus so if you have a big test coming up or a big work thing, this will really help you focus.
- It improves the quality of sleep. You will go to sleep faster when taking Ashwaganda.
- Ashwaganda is great for people who have anxiety and depression as a person with anxiety myself, I could say this herb really works because I have really bad anxiety as well as panic attacks. I haven't had one panic attack or anything since I have been taking this herb, not even a thought about anything because you know when you have anxiety you are thinking about a million things at once, but with Ashwaganda, you don't think about anything, and that's the main reason why a lot of women out here are taking it.
- Also, ladies, it helps booster fertility so be careful taking it if you don't want any kids… I would recommend taking this in the evening before you go to sleep at night so you can have a restful sleep.

Herb 5: Sea Buckthorn

The reason sea buckthorn is a great herb for women is because it contains beneficial vitamins:
It contains Antioxidants.
It also contains Fatty acids.
Additionally, Sea buckthorn oil benefits may include benefits that help with vaginal dryness if you have a problem dryness down there.

Sea Buckthorn

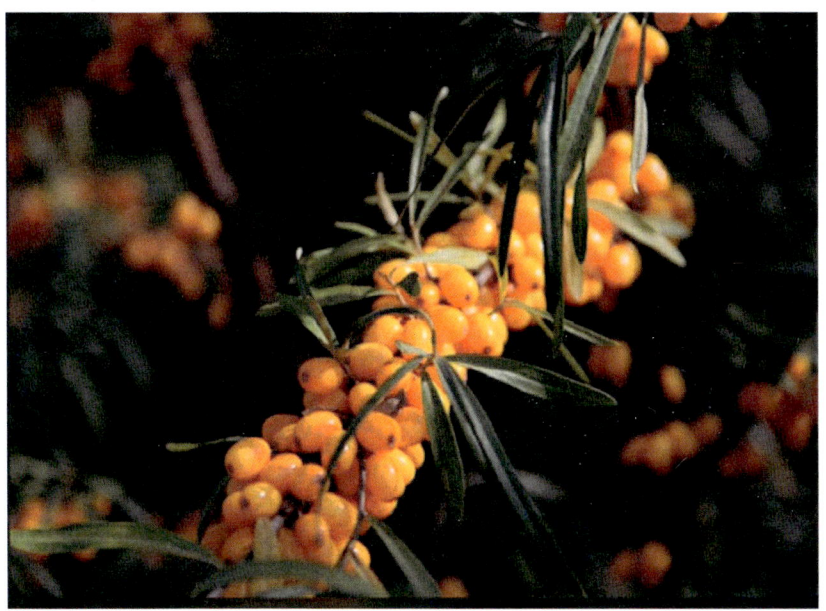

Dong Quai

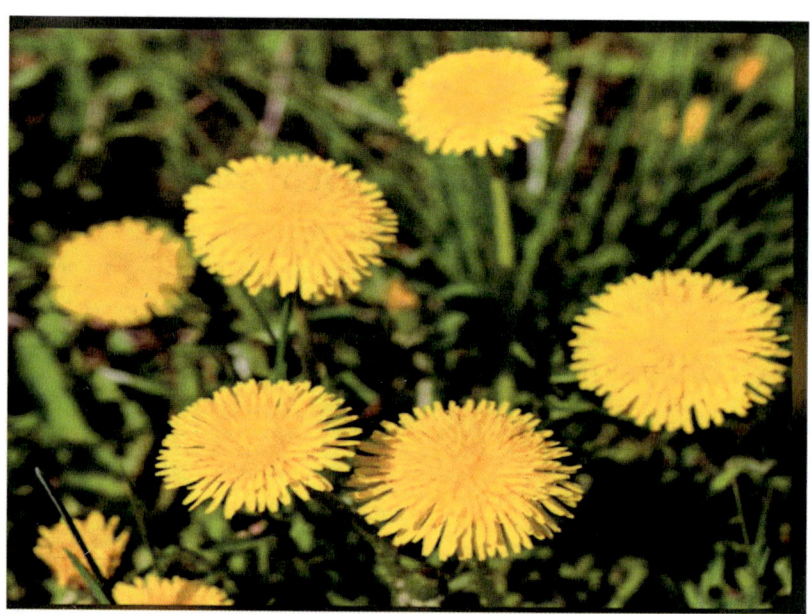

Herb 6: Dong Quai

The reason why I think that Dong quai is a great herb for women is that Dong quai is used to assist women in a number of ways such as:
- It improves blood circulation.
- It is helpful for women with menstrual problems like PMS (pre-menstrual syndrome).

Herb 6: Dong Quai continued

- It addresses cramping.
- It assists in reducing bloating.
- It improves mood swings.
- It is helpful for women with irregular periods when it is due to a weakened uterus.
- Dong quai maintains hormone balance.
- It helps regulate estrogen levels in the body whether they are too high or too low.

Not only that ladies… Dong quai also acts as a natural aphrodisiac. Studies have shown that Dong quai can increase male and female libido levels in addition to addressing issues with their fertility, so instead of going to expensive fertility centers, just try some Dong quai. You may not need to spend thousands of dollars to conceive, just by adding the powerful herb into your diet; Dong quai might help you boost your chances of conception!

Herb 7: Black Cohosh

Black cohosh is a great herb for women going through menopause because it prevents:
- Experiencing hot flashes.
- Living with night sweats.
- Enduring episodes of Vaginal dryness.
- Sleep disturbances.
- Irritability.

Additionally... Black cohosh also helps with other elements:
- Experiencing chronic anxiety.
- Dealing with bouts or constant insomnia in all women.
- It reduces the risk of blood clots and heart attacks.
- It strengthens uterine wall muscle and helps prevent miscarriages.
- It will also help with period cramps.
- It manages pain and labor contractions,
  - **but NOTE... don't drink this early in your pregnancy... drink it 3 days prior to your due date.**

- It also helps with bloating.
- It helps with morning sickness.
- It reduces flatulence.

Black Cohosh

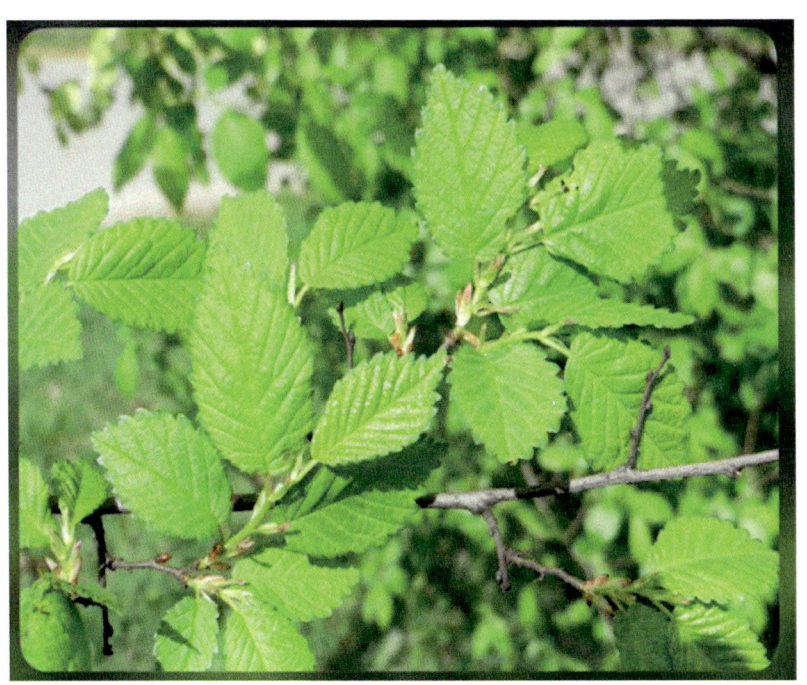

Dandelion

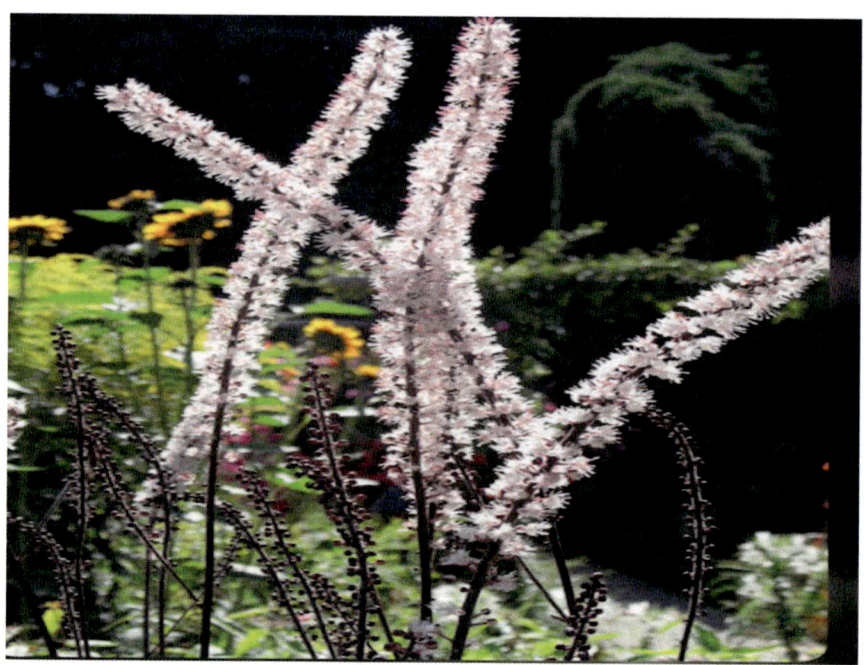

Herb 8: Dandelion

This is a good herb for women for the following reasons:
- It helps treat stomach problems.
- It helps with appendicitis.
- It helps with breast problems such as inflammation or lack of milk flow.
- It helps detox your liver.
- It helps you slow down aging.
- It also protects your skin against the sunlight and may contain anti-cancer properties.

Herb 9: Slippery Elm

Slippery elm is a great herb because it helps boost your fertility for those struggling with getting pregnant. It also helps with:
- It boosts your Libo.
- It helps with vaginal dryness which is why it is so popular among women now.
- Slippery elm is not *only good* for that it also helps with treating a sore throat.
- It helps with inflammatory bowel disease as it reduces the inflammation.
- If you are struggling with a Urinary Tract Infection, (UTI) Slippery elm helps reduce the irritation of the urinary tract ladies.

Slippery Elm

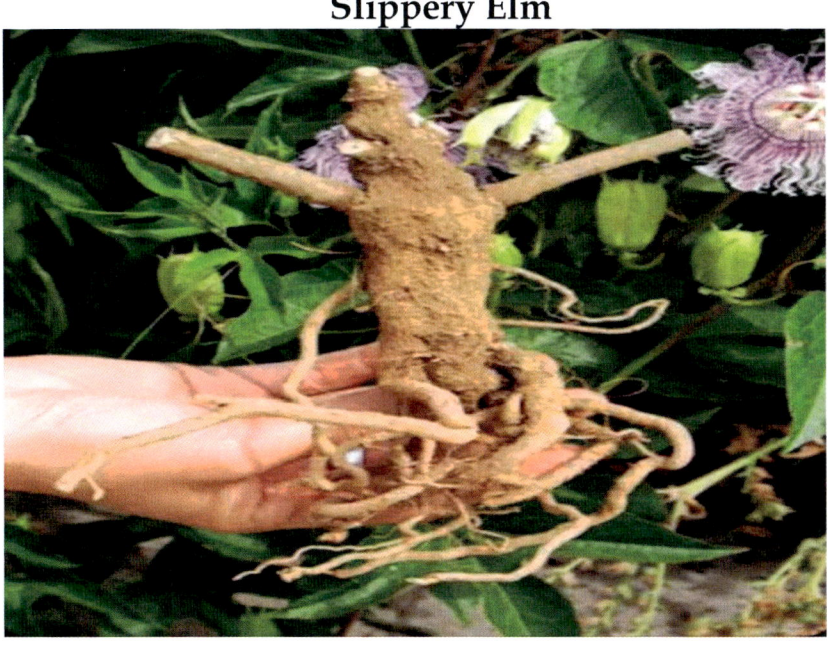

Create a woman's health plan for yourself to get you through your medical journey...

Health Plan continued...

The End!

I am Alize...
Healing myself naturally!

Hey! My name is Alize and I'm an 18-year-old girl from New York... I used herbs as natural medicine and as a way to heal myself, but *anyways*, let's get to it... the reason why I got so into herbs was because when I was 16, I got diagnosed with *Hypothyroidism*. I started having weird symptoms like heart palpitations, staying up all night, sleeping all day, losing, and gaining weight sporadically, and being extra tired. I also had an increase in anxiety resulting in fast heart rate, but not only that, it messed with my period. This issue started making my period come on at different times as well as being super painful and causing a very heavy menstrual flow.

I realized in this journey that our reproductive system can have problems and cause many women issues like having miscarriages. After going through so much I started looking for herbs that would be great for women's reproductive systems, including mine. I'm going to *make another thyroid!* I don't know when, but all I can tell y'all ladies is all I can do is try to find which herbs are helpful for women. Remember this is only some of the herb's ladies... but *anyways* using herbs are much better for your bodies than using the "stuff" doctors are trying to give us!

Made in the USA
Columbia, SC
07 August 2023